PINK
HAT
DIARIES®

Candis Low with Lisa Lively

Acknowledgements

With special thanks to…

Our families, Bill, Jordan, Savannah,
Dorothy, Carroll, Sarah, Billy, Shelley
and Ima; June, Edd, and Karen
for their love and support.

Our models, Lauren and baby Brylee.

Stan, Jeanne, Phyllis, Albert and Stephanie
for their generosity.

Betsy, for her creative design.

Rozanne and Joan for their encouragement,
friendship, and their leadership in the fight
against breast cancer.

PINK HAT DIARIES®

For information, address:
Low/Lively Productions
2000 E. Lamar Blvd., Suite 600,
Arlington, TX 76006

First low/lively productions edition:
September 2000

DEDICATION

*Dedicated to Pink Hats and their families,
and to all those who have worked so
valiantly to eradicate breast cancer
as a life-threatening disease.*

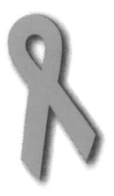

A contribution from your purchase of this book
will be made to breast health programs
and breast cancer research.

CONTENTS

FOREWORD

PINK HAT DIARIES will take you on a powerful emotional journey shared by women of all ages, ethnicity and cultures who are confronted with breast cancer. Page by page, the author and photographer portray the experiences of those whose outward badge of courage is a pink hat, worn by millions of breast cancer survivors throughout the world who participate in fund-raising events for breast cancer. To breast cancer survivors, their families, friends and supporters, pink hats are the universal symbol of breast cancer survival, representing hope for the future, and standing for the amazing strength and courage, dignity and grace of women with breast cancer.

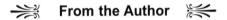

From the Author

When I reached my fourth year as a breast cancer survivor, my inspiration to write about the incredible experiences shared by so many women like me took the form of a pink hat. I wrote the stories and Lisa Lively gave birth to their universal interpretation through the eye of her camera lens.

Our goal is to reach women throughout the world who face a diagnosis of breast cancer. Our mission is to raise awareness and funds for breast cancer research.

Hopefully, in some small way, proceeds from the sale of PINK HAT DIARIES will spare our daughters and the daughters of future generations from ever having to face breast cancer.

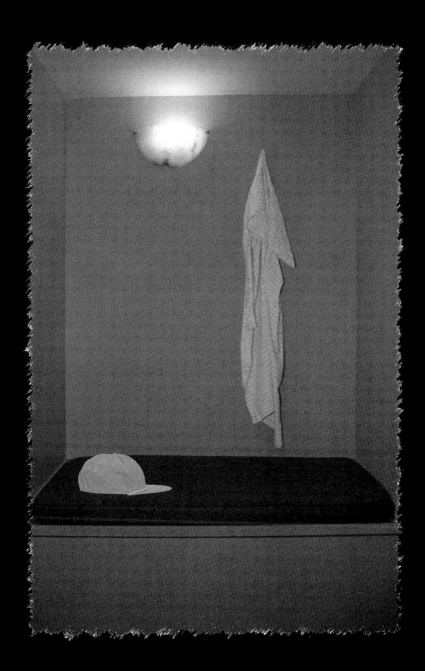

THREE

Pink Hat in Waiting

My potential
for becoming a
Pink Hat
never occurred
to me as
I sat shivering
in a thin gown
on a hard bench
in a little room
one afternoon
in the early spring
of 1996.

I hoped
the radiologist
reviewing
the image
of my breast
was giving me
an A-plus
on my
mammography
test.

I hoped
they would
politely
send me
on my way

promising
to see me
next year.

Instead,
they sent
for more tests
and eventually
told me
I had
Pink Hat
potential,
which meant
that I had
a good chance
of surviving
breast cancer.

And with those
words, my life
and the
lives of the
people
who loved me
changed
inextricably
and
forever.

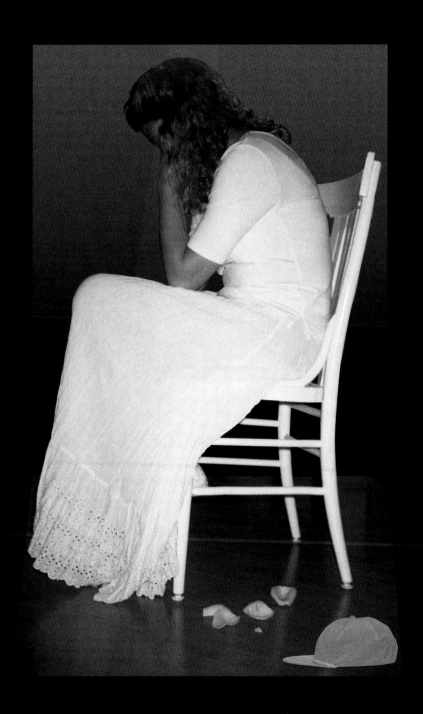

SEVEN

Pink Hat Hot List

Just who
will I tell first?
I need
to make a list.
My head
is spinning
I'm losing
touch.
I'm not
prepared
for this!

Excuse me,
friends and family,
I don't mean
to ruin your day.
Bad news,
I have breast cancer,
And oh,
by the way

Could you care
for my children?
Clean my house
and pay the bills?
I might be gone
for very long.
I've heard
that cancer kills.

If I could wake up
from this nightmare
I would spare you
from the rest
In the meantime
I'm so sorry
For the tumor
in my breast.

I need to list
my options
And the things
I have to do
Get the prayer
chain going
I'll need an extra
prayer or two.

To help me
on this journey
There is something
you can do
Just give me
love and friendship
and God
will see me through.

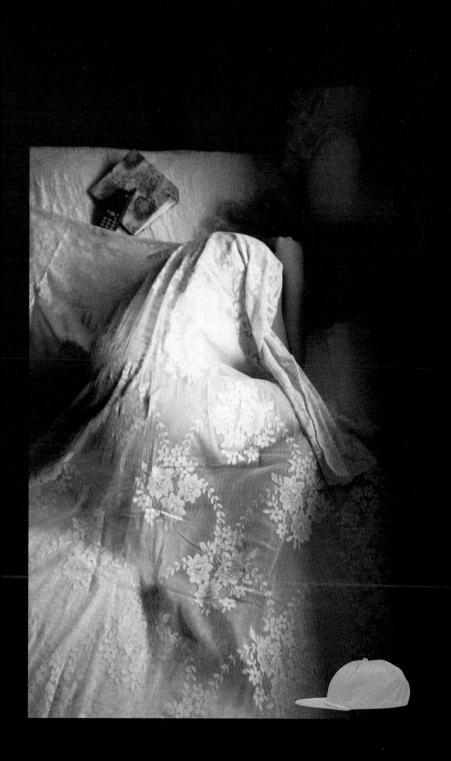

ELEVEN

Pink Hat in the Dark

Underneath
the covers
Underneath
the brave smile
and can-do attitude

In the dark
screams
ascending
from the recesses
of my inner being
crying, No!
asking, Why?
Mourning
yesterday's
invincibility
and fearing
what tomorrow
will bring.

As my husband
sleeps beside me
as my children
sleep down the hall
I weep silently
so they
cannot hear
me.

My heart
cracking
wide open
spilling tears
on sheets
the color
of eggshells
replaying words
over and over
again and again
BREAST CANCER
Under a blanket
of darkness where
the whole world
can't see
what is
just beneath
the surface
of a strong and brave
woman, mother and wife.

Only God hears
my silent screams
in the dark as
I find comfort
in prayer.

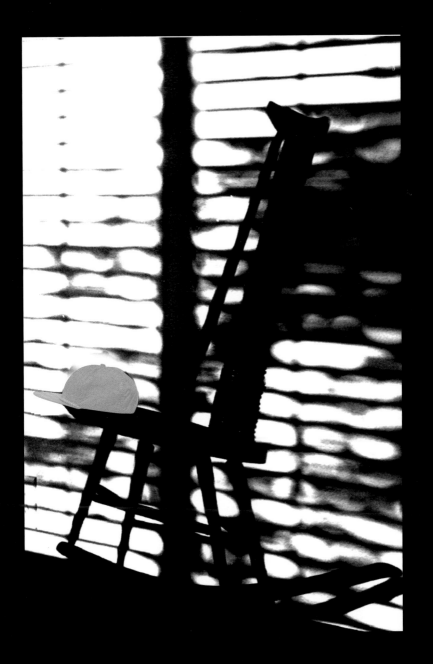

FIFTEEN

Pink Hats and Their Mothers

Standing
next to my
teenage son
dressed in black
unable
to comfort him
in his sorrow
as they lower
my body
into the ground.

I awake
shaking with fright
as I creep
from our bed
and reach
for the phone
in the early hours
of the morning.

Desperately
needing to hear
the voice
of my childhood
as I draw myself up
into a ball
on an empty chair.

Fear
sticks in my throat
like peanut butter
with no jelly
and melts away
When she says
hello.

Her voice
envelopes me
like a warm cocoon
holding me in
the safety of her
loving arms.

"Mommy,
I don't want
to die"
My voice
rises up
from the child
within
and I know
the moment
she speaks
everything
will be
alright.

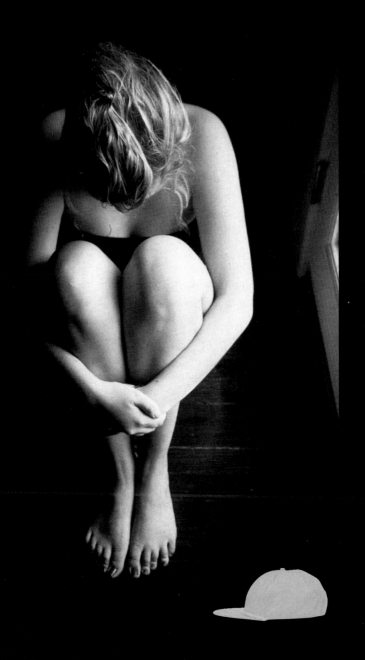

Pink Hats and Their Lovers

What will
he think?
What will
he do?
How will
things change?
Can she
get through?

What would
she look like
In the bright light?
Would he turn
the other way?

What if passion
dies
of disfigurement
And he doesn't
want to stay?

She's heard
the sad, sad stories
of the men who
just can't face
the scars of life
still healing
underneath a
sheath of lace.

She knows
he isn't like that
He doesn't love her
just for her looks
Such a small part
of the package
and not nearly
what it took

She holds
her breast
And begins
to grieve
Young lover's
vows
now under
siege

For better or worse
For richer or poorer
In sickness and in health
'Til death do us part.
Please take my breast
but not my heart

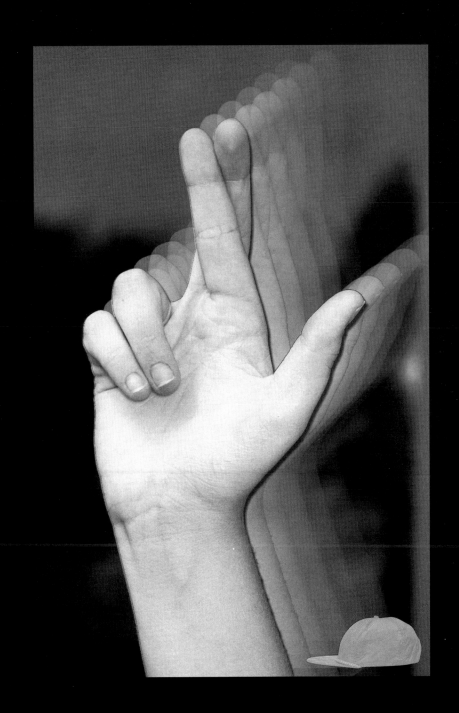

TWENTYthree

Pink Hats,
Hard Choices

Mastectomy
or Lumpectomy?
Chemotherapy
or Radiation?
Tumor Size
and to my surprise
new techniques
in reconstruction.

Chance of survival
New drug trial
Infiltrating
stage two
cancer
Statisticians
weighing
decisions
Asking questions
with no straight
answers.

It's a gamble
as I scramble
extreme measures
seem
the best
while rewriting
the final chapter

of this mystery
inside my chest.

Crossing fingers
hope life lingers
While I sign a
living will
Chemical warfare
for my welfare
hurry before
this cancer
kills.

Break out the IV's
and if you will, please
I'll take a dose of
something
light
Don't make it too strong
It might last too long
to tuck my children
in at night.

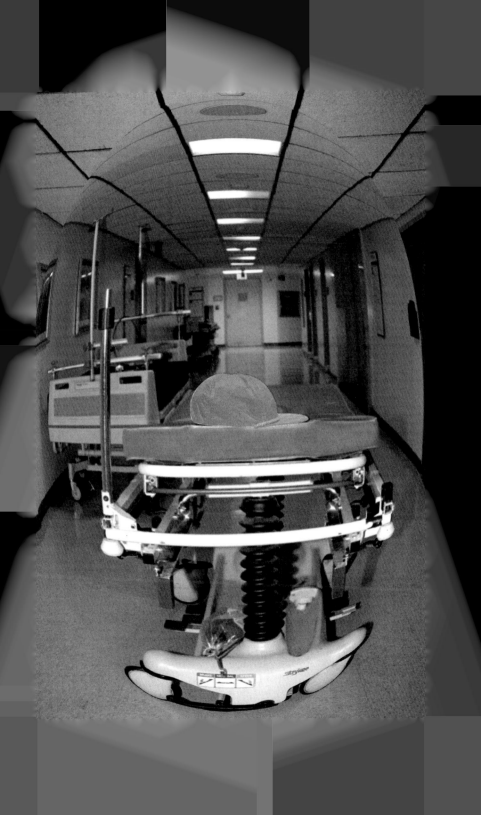

Pink Hat Walking

Walking
down the
corridor
to the prep room
where I change into
a green surgical gown
and remove my
jewelry and makeup
in slow motion
needing a few more
minutes to compose
myself in prayer
catching my reflection
one last time
in the mirror
as I undress
unable
to imagine
what will happen
next
when I take a ride
down the corridor
on a gurney
to pre-op
where plastic surgeons
with magic markers
draw pictures
on my chest

directions
for the surgeon on
the removal
of my breast.

IV dripping
reality slipping
as I begin to drift
out of consciousness
sensing a presence
I fight heavy lids to see
who has come to me
on my way to eternity.

I can barely hear
my husband speak
eyes full of love
and pain
lips whispering
my name
saying
I Love You best
His tears dripping
down
on my surgical
gown
Melting
magic marker
on my breast.

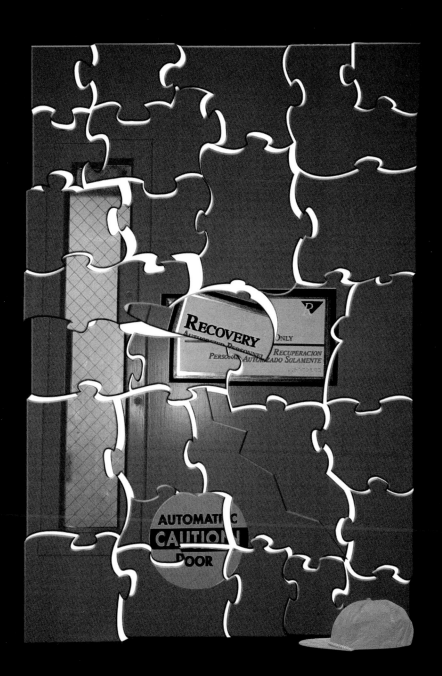

Pink Hat in Recovery

Waking up after surgery
in a place called Recovery
is full of irony
and a hard name
to put on such
a small space
when
Recovery
is a process
most Pink Hats
spend the rest
of their lives
working through.

Pink Hats waking up
in a place called
Recovery
to a different body
and a new perspective
where everything
has changed
and the promise
of tomorrow
lingers
in their attitudes
about a process
whose label
is a sign on the door
of the first room
they enter
after surgery.

Pink Hats
picking up
the pieces
in Recovery
after science
and medicine
exact their price
and
leave them
to their own
devices.

Pink Hats
rise
to the
occasion
blending
doses
of religion,
friends
and family
self love
and spirituality
into medicine
that begins
where
science
leaves off
on their
lifelong
journey to
Recovery.

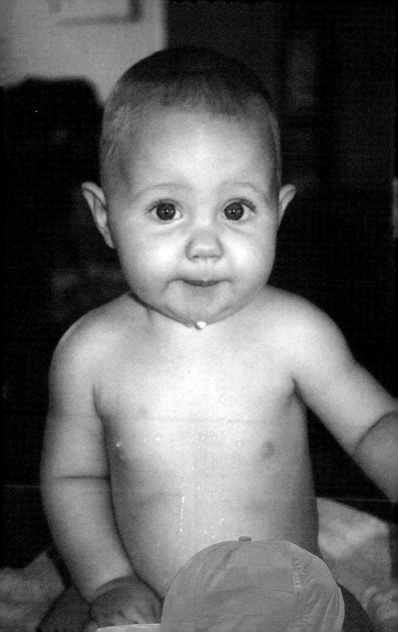

Pink Hats, Bald Heads

Bald heads
like billboards
announce their plight
Pink Hats
courageously
poised for the fight

Pink Hats
determined
to get on with
their lives
mothers, daughters,
sisters and wives

Spying a Pink Hat
I feel so inclined
to share my
happy ending
while standing in line

"Hello," I say,
"I made it,
and so will you…
my hair grew back curly
yours will, too!"

I listen
as she tells me
her cancer has spread
while she smiles
and pats her smooth bald head.

She hugs me
and whispers
under her breath,
"It's good to know
I might cheat death…"

"But there's
so much more
to do today
than think about
my lost toupee"

"I want to
live and love
while I still can,
I'm engaged to marry
a wonderful man!"

"I'll be
twenty three
on the fifth of June
I just can't leave
It's much too soon"

I nod my head
and walk away
thankful
there is
so much
more
to do today.

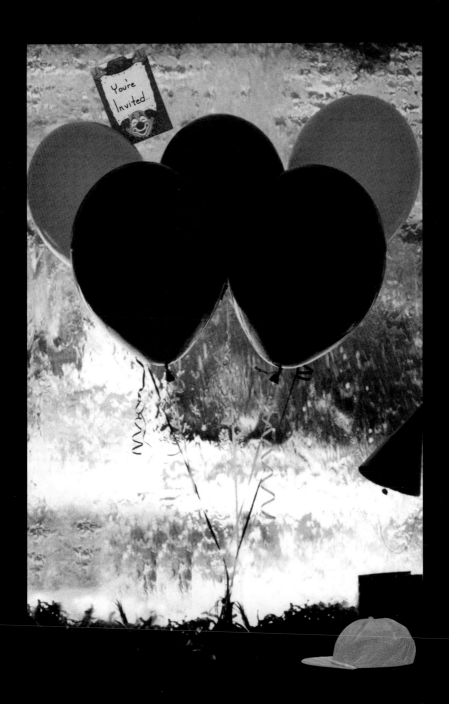

Pink Hat on a Bad Day

Bring on the
pity party
and let me
have my way
to do nothing but
feel sorry for
my sad sick self
all day.

After all, I know
I deserve to cry
and wallow in
my pain
So bring on
the pity party
and I'll show
you what I mean.

Give me
a box of tissues
and some pictures
of back then
I want to mourn
my losses and get rid
of all this phlegm
Just when
I think it's over
it wells up in me again.

I need to purge
the hurt and fear
so please just be
a friend.

Break out
the pity party
Let my eyes
get really red
Don't tell me
crying doesn't help
Without it
I'd be dead.

Some day
I won't require
a pity party
every week
perhaps a
monthly cleansing
of which
I'll seldom speak.

But just for now
have faith in me
and no,
I'm not depressed
It's an ancient
form of therapy
that women
do best.

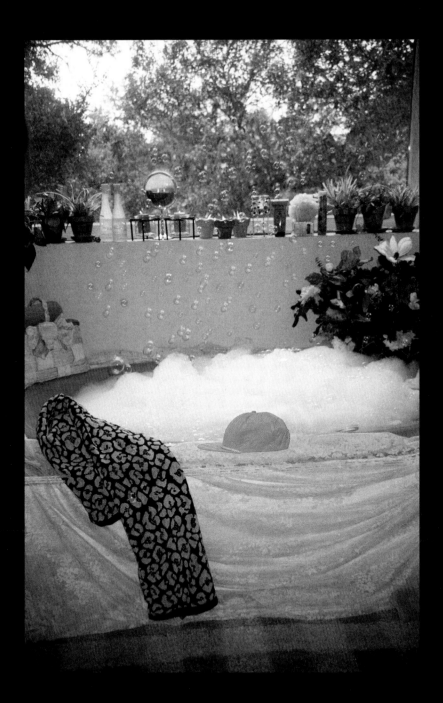

Pink Hat in the Bathtub

Bubbling with delight
at discovering
Mommy in the bathtub
she begs to join me
while flinging her clothes
this way and that
and before I can say
"not this time"
she is in the tub
splashing and giggling in a tidal wave
of warm sudsy water
washing away
my bubble bra
with her enthusiastic arrival.

I draw my knees up to hide my chest
but not soon enough
to keep her from seeing
the angry red scars
instead of the breast
that nurtured her
just two years ago.

Horrified, I hold my breath
as she asks in a curious tone,
"Mommy, what's that?"
with a chubby finger
outstretched as if pointing
to an unfamiliar vegetable
on her dinner plate.

With the precision
of a seasoned actor
delivering her lines
I put on my mommy voice
and gently reply,
"Mommy had a bad booboo
and the doctor cut it out."

"Oh." She responds casually,
while crossing her eyes
and reaching forward
to pop a bubble as it settles
on the tip of her outstretched finger.

I can feel more questions lingering
like little bubbles waiting to be burst.
"Mommy, can you still run after me?"
she asks, throwing her arms around me.
Laughing hysterically,
I kiss her cheek and say,
"Yes, sweetie, I can run faster than ever."

I look at her with profound love,
and while marveling at her logic,
I feel so very blessed.
Yes, my darling daughter
You are so right.
I don't need my breast
to chase you and catch you.
I don't need my breast
to be the best mommy in the world.

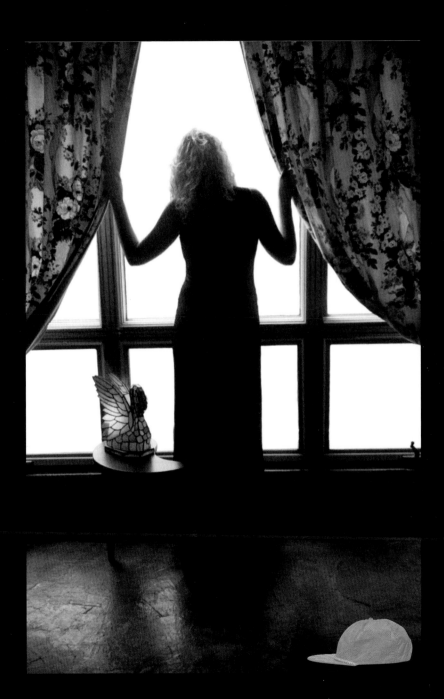

Pink Hat with a Sense of Sensuality

Competitors
are now
admirers

Thinking
their men
are safe with me
Since I lost
my thirty-six
double-d

When underneath
most explicitly
lies a dormant
sensuality

Tempered by
the surgeon's knife
still reeling from
the fight for life

It will awake
in time
desire
and light
long sleeping
passion's fire

My strength
courage
faith and
dignity

Hold
far more
sensuality
than any
thirty-six
double-d

Driven by
a power
within
appealing to
the souls of
men

So hold
on to your
bras
and I'll
hold on
to my hat.
A sexy
pink hat…
Imagine that!

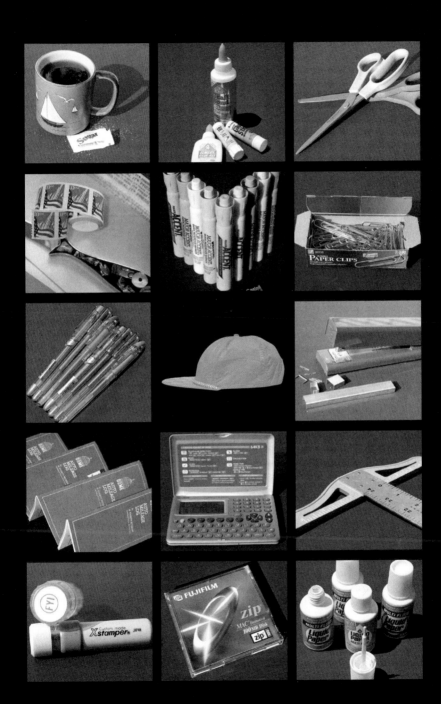

Pink Hat in the Workplace

Do people
in the workplace
treat Pink Hats
differently?

I think about
my colleagues
and wonder
what their
reaction will be.

Will they
still want to
work with me?

When I find
the courage
to tell them
I wipe away
the tears of many
caring people.

I see a lot of pain
and hear their
stories
of wives, mothers,
sisters and daughters
with breast cancer;
some who survived
and some who died.

They may not know it
but they give me
courage that day.

They tell me
they believed
I could beat it.
They tell me
I have what it takes
to win my battle.
They tell me
I inspire them.
They make me
stronger
and more
determined
than ever.

I know
that if they ever
have to draw from
my experience,
I want them
to gain strength
from having known me.
If I can serve
as a reminder
to remember
the importance of
early detection,
then somehow,
I can make sense
of what was happening.

I return to work
after surgery,
still taking rounds
of chemotherapy.

IV connected to a
shunt in my arm
I roll my IV stand
to the nurses station
to use the telephone.

Conducting
business
as usual,
calendar
in one hand,
phone perched
on my shoulder
while making notes
and taking orders.

I turn
to notice
all eyes
in the oncology lab
are on me.
I can't resist
the temptation,
and break out
in song…
"If they could
see me now,
those customers of mine…"

A hush falls over
the room
while all at once
tired eyes
narrow and
begin to sparkle
as if every
funnybone
in their bodies
struck the same
chord
and they begin
to laugh.

The laughter
in the
oncology lab
today
probably
kills
more
cancer cells
than
chemotherapy
drugs
ever could.

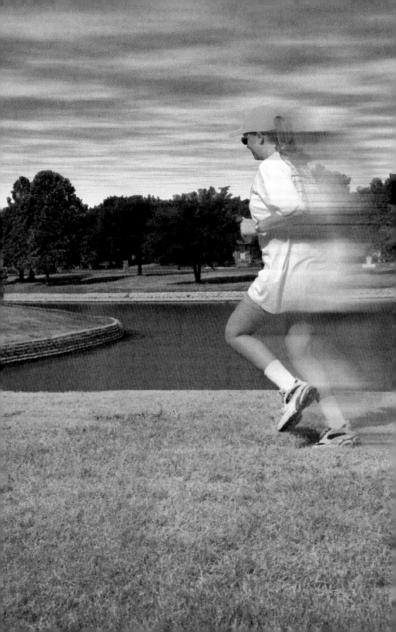

Pink Hat Racing

Three months
into forty-nine
laugh lines
and cry lines
gray hairs
and stray hairs
one less breast
but who cares.

Alive and well,
so far so good
didn't die
thought I could
my hat is pink
my hair is thin
a casualty of
the war within.

A body scarred
the cost of life
still a beloved
mom and wife
walking among
so many like me
thankful to
be cancer free.

Kindred spirits
soul searching eyes
been there looks
with no disguise
there are no strangers
in this place
Pink Hats together
running the race.

A race for life
a race for the cure
so many lost
so much endured
Pink Hats like medals
from the fight
On heads of heroes,
An awesome sight.

PINK
HAT
DIARIES

Candis Low with Lisa Lively

Pink Hat
with Attitude

There are strangers
who treat us differently
when they find out
we've had
a mastectomy
and we can predict
with accuracy
exactly what
their reaction
is going to be.

Words laced
with subtle
innuendoes
while wishing us
their best
when they think
we're not looking
they're staring
at our chests.

Their eyes mirror
true feelings
veiled with
vanity and pride
through the pretense
of acceptance
we sense fear
deep down inside.

Fear
of getting cancer
through
just knowing
it exists
might move them
to do something
to eliminate
their risk

So if our recent
struggle
with the
deadliest disease
makes you a bit
uncomfortable
then pardon us
but please

Go get yourself
a mammogram
and tell a friend
or two
because before
you know it
the next
Pink Hat
could be
you!

ABOUT THE AUTHOR...

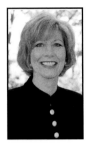 An accomplished writer and public relations consultant, PINK HAT DIARIES author Candis Low demonstrates her craft in the art of communicating with frankness and sensitivity. A four year survivor of breast cancer, Candis is actively involved in volunteer work, serving as a member of the Tarrant County Affiliate Board of Directors of the Susan G. Komen Breast Cancer Foundation, and as Public Relations Chair for the Tarrant County, Texas Komen Race for the Cure®. As a recipient of the 1999 Komen Spirit Award, Candis represented her affiliate at the National Race for the Cure® in Washington, D.C., where she was honored by Al and Tipper Gore at the Vice President's residence. Candis Low lives in Arlington, Texas with her husband, Bill, and children, Jordan and Savannah.

ABOUT THE PHOTOGRAPHER...

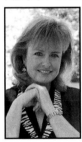 The many faces, landscapes and cultures of five continents prepared Lisa Lively for the technical and artistic challenges that this book demanded. A native Texan and Fine Arts graduate of Texas Christian University, Lisa spent eighteen years as an Advertising Account Executive before taking time off to portray the deep feelings described in PINK HAT DIARIES. Her intimate photographs have faithfully documented the exhaustive range of emotions that temporarily shattered the life of her friend – the strong and valiant author of this diary. Lisa chose black and white film to complement the moods of the diary as the layers of fear and anguish gradually peeled away to expose the brilliant light that lies sheltered within each human heart.

To Order Additional Copies Of

PINK HAT DIARIES®

Call Toll Free

1-866-PinkHat

Visit Our Website at
www.pinkhatdiaries.com

We Would Love To Hear From You!
Email: pinkhatdiaries@yahoo.com